MW01234958

The Holistic Guide to Wellness

Discover Natural Herbal Remedies for Limitless Health

ISBN 978-1-300-79860-6
Tony Biermann
Copyright@2024

TABLE OF CONTENT

CHAPTER 1 3
  INTRODUCTION 3
CHAPTER 2 9
  Understanding Holistic Wellness9
CHAPTER 3 16
  The Power of Natural Herbal
  Remedies 16
CHAPTER 4 23
  Key Herbal Remedies for
  Common Ailments 23
CHAPTER 5 56
  Preparing and Using Herbal
  Remedies 56
THE END 63

CHAPTER 1

INTRODUCTION

Describes holistic wellness.

In the search of ideal well-being, holistic wellness—body, mind, and spirit—consumes the whole individual. Unlike conventional medicine, which sometimes concentrates on treating certain symptoms or diseases, holistic wellness stresses the connectivity of all elements of an individual's life and strives to foster balance and harmony. This method acknowledges that physical health cannot be totally attained without also attending to emotional, psychological, and spiritual well-being.

Important ideas guiding holistic wellness consist in:

Combining alternative therapies including acupuncture, chiropractic treatment, and herbal therapy with traditional medicine yields integration of many health practices.

Encouragement of people to actively participate in preserving their health by means of lifestyle decisions, self-care, and preventative actions comes under personal responsibility.

Prevention Over Cure: Giving long-term health top priority instead of just treating diseases means giving techniques that prevent disease top priority.

Treating patients as unique people with different needs and preferences rather than using a one-size-fits-all strategy is known as patient-centered care.

Value in Herbal and Natural Remedies

For millennia, many civilizations all around have employed natural and herbal treatments to preserve health and cure diseases. For people looking for substitutes for manufactured medications, these remedies—derived from plants and natural sources—appealingly seem. Natural and herbal medicines are important as their many advantages define them.

Many herbal cures have less adverse effects than synthetic medications. For instance, chamomile tea is well-known for its relaxing properties free of the dependency problems related to several prescription sleep aids.

Often more reasonably priced than pharmaceutical drugs are herbal medicines. Growing your own medical plants might help to lower expenses even more.

Natural cures are commonly obtained in local health food stores, farmers' markets, or even your own backyard and are rather accessible.

Using natural medicines usually requires less industrial processing and less resources, so they might be more ecologically friendly.

Herbal medicine offers a continuity and link to ancient practices since it is firmly ingrained in many civilizations and traditions.

Advantages of a whole-hearted approach to health

Enhanced Physical Health: Holistic wellness can result in greater general physical health by means of treating the underlying causes of health problems and advocating preventive actions. Including regular physical activity, a balanced diet, and enough sleep, for instance, helps avoid obesity, heart disease, and diabetes.

Improved Emotional and Mental Well-Being: Holistic wellness values mental and emotional wellness. Mindfulness, meditation, and counseling among other techniques assist people control depression, anxiety, and stress, so enhancing mental clarity and emotional resilience.

Holistic wellness sees every person as unique and offers individualized care regimens catered to their particular requirements and preferences. This method helps people to better understand their body and psyche, so enabling them to make wise medical decisions.

Strengthened Immune System: Natural therapies and lifestyle choices that strengthen the immune system are sometimes part of a complete treatment. Eating a diet high in minerals, vitamins, and antioxidants from fruits and vegetables, for instance, helps strengthen immune system and lower disease risk.

Holistic wellness stresses the need of controlling stress by means of yoga, meditation, deep breathing exercises, and aromatherapy among other approaches. Good stress management helps to avoid the detrimental consequences of ongoing stress on mental and physical health.

Unlike only treating symptoms, holistic wellness seeks to heal the entire person. Since the fundamental causes of health problems are resolved, this can lead to more significant and long-lasting benefits for health.

A whole approach promotes a balanced lifestyle with good diet, frequent exercise, enough relaxation, and deep social contacts. A more content and fulfilling existence can result from this equilibrium.

Holistic wellness helps people to take control of their health and develop more self-awareness. Better health decisions and a closer awareness of one's own needs and limitations can follow from this self-awareness.

Holistic wellness offers a more complete approach to health and can enhance traditional medical therapies. To improve their efficacy and lower adverse effects, for instance, herbal supplements or acupuncture might be used in addition to traditional treatments.

Holistic wellness supports long-term maintenance of sustainable health practices by means of which one can This

covers developing good habits that fit
one's way of life rather than only
transient solutions.

CHAPTER 2

Understanding Holistic Wellness

Definitions and Holistic Health's Principles

In the search of ideal health and well-being, holistic health—which integrates the mind, body, and spirit—considers the full person. Unlike conventional medicine, which sometimes concentrates on treating certain symptoms or diseases, holistic health stresses the interconnectivity of all elements of an individual's life and strives to foster balance and harmony.

Important tenets of holistic health consist in:

Holistic health mixes alternative therapies such yoga, herbal medicine, chiropractic care, and acupuncture with traditional medical treatments. This combined strategy offers a more all-encompassing way of handling medical issues.

Holistic health views each person as unique and with different requirements and preferences. Emphasizing individualized treatment plans catered to

each person's particular situation, this method takes physical, emotional, psychological, and spiritual aspects into account.
Holistic health stresses proactive steps to sustain health rather than only treating problems. This covers frequent exercise, good diet, stress management, and visits to identify possible problems early on.

People are urged to actively participate in their health and well-being by self-care and responsibility. This covers choosing a diet, exercise, sleep schedule, and stress-reducing strategy as well as obtaining suitable medical attention as needed.

Holistic health stresses the need of reaching harmony and balance in every sphere of life. This covers physical, psychological, emotional, and spiritual wellness. One can reach this equilibrium by means of practices including meditation, mindfulness, and relaxation strategies.

Rather than concentrating just on symptoms, holistic healing seeks to treat the underlying causes of medical problems. Usually, this method produces more significant and long-lasting changes in general health.

Holistic health acknowledges the strong interaction between the body and the mind. Physical health can be much influenced by emotional and psychological states; vice versa. For general health, then, mental and emotional well-being is absolutely vital.

the Mind-Body Link

Emphasizing the link between mental, emotional, and physical well-being, the basic idea in holistic health is the mind-body connection. Achieving whole wellbeing requires an awareness of this relationship.

Psychological Effects on Physical Health: Directly influencing physical health are emotions and mental states. Chronic stress, for instance, can cause digestive problems, lowered immune system, and high blood pressure. On the other hand, mental moods and pleasant emotions can support physical health and healing.

Physical Health Affecting Mental Well-Being: Moreover affecting mental and emotional well-being are physical health problems. For instance, illnesses or persistent pain can cause worry, sadness, and frustration. Dealing with physical health problems might help one to develop both mentally and emotionally.

The mind-body link is demonstrated by the body's reaction to stress and relaxation. Fight or flight reaction triggered by chronic stress raises blood pressure, heart rate, and cortisol levels. Over time, this can compromise health. Deep breathing, meditation, and yoga among other relaxation techniques can set off the rest and digest reaction, therefore fostering healing and peace.

Practices that help to strengthen the mind-body connection are mindfulness and meditation. These techniques center on the here and now and help one develop nonjudging awareness of ideas and feelings. Regular meditation and mindfulness help to lower stress, increase mental clarity, and foster emotional resilience.

Emotional Release and Physical Healing: Physical healing can follow from emotional release of tension. Talk therapy, journaling, and expressive arts are among the tools available to assist people process and release emotional tension, therefore enhancing their physical condition.

The mind-body connection can be improved with several holistic therapies including chiropractic care, massage, and acupuncture. Often addressing both physical and mental aspects of health, these therapies support general well-being.

The Part Lifestyle Choices Play in Holistic Wellness

Holistic wellness depends much on lifestyle choices. People can greatly affect their general health and well-being by changing bad habits and choosing wisely. Important lifestyle choices include:

Holistic wellness depends on a balanced and nouraging diet. A range of entire foods—fruits, vegetables, whole grains, lean meats, and good fats—supplies the essential nutrients for best health. Steer clear of processed foods, too much sugar, and bad fats to help boost vitality and prevent chronic diseases.

Maintaining physical health, lowering risk of chronic diseases, and enhancing mental well-being all depend on consistent physical activity. A well-rounded fitness program can be created by combining aerobic exercise, strength training, flexibility exercises, and activities encouraging relaxation—like yoga and tai chi.

Enough sleep and rest are absolutely vital for general health. Among the several health problems poor sleep can cause are compromised immune system, more stress, and worse cognitive ability. Developing a consistent sleeping schedule and designing a peaceful sleeping environment helps to enhance general well-being and quality of sleep.

Comprehensive wellness depends on the management of stress. Long-term stress can compromise mental as well as physical health. Resilience and relaxation can be fostered by including stress-reducing techniques including meditation, deep breathing exercises, gradual muscular relaxation, and time in nature.

Emotional and mental well-being depends critically on strong social ties and relationships. Good relationships lessen stress, offer support, and advance a feeling of purpose and belonging. Participating in social events, tending to current connections, and looking for encouraging communities will improve general quality of life.

A major component of holistic wellbeing is the care of mental and emotional health. This covers developing self-compassion, getting therapy or counseling if needed, establishing reasonable limits, and participating in joyful and fulfilling activities.

Personal Development and Spirituality: Personal development and spirituality can help one to find direction and meaning in life. This can entail investigating personal values, creating goals, practicing spirituality, or following hobbies and activities consistent with one's passions and convictions.

Practicing mindfulness and living in the moment will help one to improve their general state of health. Mindfulness is the ability to pay attention to the current moment free from judgment, so helping to lower stress, increase mental clarity, and strengthen bonds with people and oneself.

Maintaining general heath depends on consistent self-care routines. This covers leisure, introspection, and self-nurturing pursuits including bathing, reading, artistic projects, and time spent in the natural world.

CHAPTER 3

The Power of Natural Herbal Remedies

Herbal Medicine's Origins and History

Among the first known forms of medication used by humans is herbal medicine, sometimes referred to as botanical medicine or phytotherapy. Its beginnings can be seen in prehistoric societies all around, each of which created their own special system for medical use of plants.

Historic civilizations:

Ancient Egypt: Among the first to record using herbs were Egyptians. Comprising hundreds of herbal cures, the Ebers Papyrus—which dates back to about 1550 BC—is among the earliest and most thorough documentation of ancient Egyptian medical techniques.

Rooted on a philosophy stressing harmony and balance, traditional Chinese medicine (TCM) has used herbs for about 2,500 years. Among the first compilations of herbal knowledge in China is the Shennong Ben Cao Jing, Divine Farmer's Materia Medica.

Originating in India more than 3,000 years ago, Ayurveda is a holistic system of medicine based on a great range of herbs to balance the body's doshas, or energy forces. Books such as the Charaka Samhita and Sushruta Samhita go into great length on the usage of several plants for medicine.

Inspired by past civilizations, ancient Greek and Roman doctors such as Hippocrates and Galen published a great deal on the medical use of plants. For almost a millennium, Dioscorides' De Materia Medica—written in the first century AD—was the pillar of herbal knowledge in Europe.

Renaissance and Middle Ages Europe:

Monasteries developed as hubs of herbal knowledge during the Middle Ages when monks kept medicinal gardens and copied ancient books. A 12th-century abbess, Hildegard of Bingen wrote a great deal on herbs' medicinal uses.

Herbal medicine revived attention throughout the Renaissance as figures like Paracelsus promoted the use of plants depending on their signatures, or resemblances to body parts.

Native Customs:

Rich herbal medicinal customs abound in indigenous civilizations all around. For millennia, Native American cultures have made use of herbs including echinacea and willow bark. Likewise, a variety of native flora has long been the foundation of African and Australian Aboriginal medicine.

Science Underlying Herbal Remedies

Many conventional uses of herbs have been confirmed by modern science, which has revealed their molecular pathways. Herbal medicine is the study of the complicated interactions among the several chemicals present in plants.

Active compounds are:

Alkaloids: Strong physiological effects abound from nitrogen-containing substances. One strong pain reliever, for instance, morphine from the opium poppy (Papaver somniferum).

Antioxidant qualities of flavonoids are well established. Common in many fruits and vegetables, flavonoids help lower inflammation and guard against chronic conditions.

Terpenes: Various medicinal effects abound in these aromatic molecules.

Menthol from peppermint (Mentha piperita) for example has analgesic and cooling properties.

Glycosides: These substances can affect the heart really significantly. Heart failure is treated with Digitalis, taken from foxglove (Digitalis purpurea).

Pharmaceutics:

Understanding how herbal ingredients interact with the body at the molecular level helps one better appreciate their benefits. For instance, turmeric's (Curcuma longa) chemical curcumin has been demonstrated to alter inflammatory pathways.

Herbal treatments frequently call for using the entire plant or a mix of plants, which can have synergistic benefits. This implies that the whole effect of all the components of a plant can be more than their individual values taken together. For instance, traditional Chinese formulations' mix of several herbs is meant to balance and maximize their benefits.

Clinical Studies:

Evidence-Based Herbal Medicine: Herbal medicines' effectiveness is being tested in ever more clinical investigations. Studies have indicated, for example, that St. John's Wort (Hypericum perforatum) can help mild to moderate depression.

Safety and Dosage: Studies on the safety and appropriate dosage of herbal treatments also abound. Therapeutic dosages must be decided upon using minimum risk of side effects or interactions with other drugs.

Typical Fallacies and Stories

Even although herbal treatment is supported by an increasing amount of scientific data, some misunderstandings and false beliefs endure. Dealing with issues enables people to make wise decisions about their health.

natural means safe:

One of the most often held false beliefs is that every natural product is intrinsically safe. Although many herbs have lengthy history of safe use, some can be poisonous or produce side effects. For instance, if handled improperly, the extremely poisonous plant aconite (Aconitum spp.) can cause major medical problems.

Natural does not always equal safe or free from side effects, hence one must realize. One needs proper knowledge and direction from a skilled practitioner.

Herbs: Pseudoscientific or ineffective

Another fallacy holds that herbal therapy has no scientific worth or potency. Many plants, though, have been well investigated and shown to have therapeutic value. For instance, well-documented are turmeric's anti-inflammatory qualities, echinacea's immune-boosting effects, and hawthorn's (Crataegus spp.) heart-supportive virtues.

Denying herbal medicine as pseudoscience ignores its possible advantages and the thorough studies backing up its usage.

Herbs Work Immediately:

Like modern medications, some people hope natural therapies would offer instant relief. Herbs, on the other hand, often act more slowly and treat the fundamental causes of medical problems instead of merely symptoms. More long-lasting and environmentally friendly outcomes can follow from this slower, more comprehensive approach.

Using herbal medicines calls for persistence and patience since their full effects may take time to develop.

One-Size-fits-all:

Herbal medicine is quite unique; what benefits one person might not help another. An individual's response to a certain plant might be influenced by body type, constitution, and unique medical conditions.

See a skilled practitioner to help customize herbal remedies to fit specific needs.

Herbs Are Only for Minor Ails:

Some people think herbs are only good for mild ailments and cannot treat more severe illnesses. Herbal medicine can help to manage chronic problems, increase general wellbeing, and improve the efficacy of conventional therapies even if it should not replace them for severe diseases.

For instance, by reducing side effects and improving general health, herbal treatments can help cancer patients on chemotherapy.

CHAPTER 4

Key Herbal Remedies for Common Ailments

Herbal remedies for stress and anxiety

Common problems influencing millions of individuals globally are stress and anxiety. Although there are several traditional therapies accessible, many people choose herbal remedies as a natural substitute to help control these disorders. Some of the most powerful herbal treatments for stress and anxiety are thoroughly explored here.

Ashwagandha (Withania somnifera)

For millennia Ayurvedic medicine has made use of the adaptogenic herb ashwagandha, sometimes referred to as Indian ginseng. Adaptogens support the body in preserving equilibrium and adjusting to stress.

Ashwagandha has been demonstrated to lower the main stress hormone in the body, cortisol. It increases general well-being, raises energy levels, and helps to ease anxiety.

Ashwagandha can be taken in capsules, powders, and tinctues among other forms. Usually, a dosage consists in 300 to 500 mg of standardized extract every day.

Generally regarded as safe for most individuals, pregnant or nursing women should avoid it. It's best to see a healthcare professional before use since it can interfere with some drugs.

Chamomile, or Matricaria chamomilla,

Overview: Renowned for its relaxing and soothing qualities, chamomile is a herb. Usually drank as a tea.

Apigenin, an antioxidant found in chamomile that hooks to certain brain receptors, helps to relax and lowers anxiety. It can also facilitate better quality of sleep.

Usually drank as a tea, chamomile is made from one to two tsp of dried flowers soaked in boiling water for five to ten minutes. One might take it three times a day.

Safety: Though it might induce allergic responses in those sensitive to daisy family plants, chamomile is usually safe.

It might potentially interact with drugs that thin blood.

Lavender, or lavandula angustifolia

Lavender is well known for its relaxing properties and pleasing scent. Herbal medicine and aromatherapy have long benefited from its use.

Lavender oil has been demonstrated to help one relax, boost mood, and lower anxiety. It also aids with sleep problems.

Lavender can be found in capsules, teas, and essential oils as well as in other forms. Few drops of lavender oil can be used to a diffuser or rubbed on the skin (diluted with a carrier oil) in aromatherapy.

Safety: Lavender is usually safe; the essential oil should not be consumed. Some people may get skin irritation from it, hence a patch test is advised before using topicals.

Valerian Root (Officinalis valerian)

Overview: From ancient times, valerian root has been utilized to help with sleep and relaxation.

Valerian root has elements that raise gamma-aminobutyric acid (GABA) in the brain, therefore soothing the nervous system and lowering stress.

Valerian root finds use in capsules, tinctures, and teas. Usually taken 30 minutes to two hours before bed, a dose ranges from 300 to 600 mg of valerian extract.

Safety: Valerian is usually safe for short-term use although some people experience stomach discomfort, headache, and vertigo. Long-term use is not advised without professional direction.

Passiflora incarnata, the passion flower

Passionflower is a climbing vine used historically to cure sleeplessness and anxiety.

Passionflower acts by raising GABA levels in the brain, therefore lowering anxiety and encouraging peace.

Consumption of passionflower might be as a pill, tincture, or tea. Usually, one takes 400 to 500 mg of standardized extract daily.

Though some people may get tiredness and dizziness, passionflower is usually safe. It shouldn't be taken in concert with sedative drugs.

Mel Melissa officinalis, lemon balm

Overview: Originally belonging to the mint family, lemon balm has been used for ages to lower stress and boost mood.

Benefits include lemon balm's relaxing effect on the nervous system, ability to assist lower anxiety, improve sleep, and boost cognitive abillty.

You might drink lemon balm as a pill, tincture, or tea. Usually, a dosage ranges from 300 to 600 mg of extract daily, or one to two teaspoons of dried leaves steeped in hot water.

Safety: Although lemon balm is usually harmless, some people get stomach pain and nausea. It might interfere with thyroid meds.

Rosea rhodiola

Rhodiola rosea is an adaptogenic herb native in hilly, cold environments. It has long been employed to improve mental and physical performance.

Rhodiola balances cortisol levels, therefore helping the body to adapt to stress. It can help to lower anxiety, raise mood, increase general vitality and resilience.

Rhodiola comes as tinctues and capsules. Usually, one takes 200 to 600 mg of standardized extract daily.

Safety: Rhodiola is usually harmless, however in some people it can induce adverse effects including dry mouth and vertigo. One should avoid taking it in the evening since it could induce sleeplessness.

Kava (Piper methysticum)

Native to the South Pacific islands, kava is a herb used historically in ceremonies to encourage restfulness.

Kava has sedative and anxiolytic properties from substances known as kavalactones. It can encourage tranquilly and aid ease anxiousness.

Kava comes as teas, pills, and tinctues. Usually, a daily dosage consists in 100 to 300 mg of kavalactones.

Safety: If taken for long periods or in great quantities, kava might harm liver

function. Following dose instructions and seeing a healthcare professional before use is absolutely vital.
Ocimum sanctum, holy basil

Known by many as tulsi, holy basil is an adaptogenic herb prized in Ayurvedic medicine for its ability to reduce stress.

Holy basil has benefits in lowering cortisol levels, raising mood, and sharpening mental sharpness. Its anti-inflammatory and antioxidant qualities also abound.

Holy basil may be taken as a pill, tincture, or tea. Usually, one takes between 300 and 500 mg of extract daily.

Safety: Although holy basil is usually harmless, some people experience side effects like nausea and diarrhea. It might mix with drugs that thin blood.

Ginseng, from Panax spp.,

Overview: For millennia people have utilized the adaptogenic herb ginseng to boost general well-being, lower stress, and increase energy.

Benefits: Through control of cortisol levels, ginseng aids in the body's stress adaptation. It can raise resilience, improve mood, and sharpen cognitive ability.

Use: Ginseng comes in drinks, pills, and powders. Usually, one takes 200 to 400 mg of standardized extract daily.

Though some people have adverse effects like headache, disturbed sleep, and gastrointestinal problems, ginseng is usually harmless. It shouldn't be taken for long stretches without medical supervision or in great quantities.

Herbs for Immune Support
Defending the body against infections, diseases, and toxins calls for a strong immune system. Although a good diet, consistent exercise, enough sleep, and stress management are absolutely vital for preserving immune system function, some herbs can give the immune system extra help. Here we look at many herbs with immune-boosting qualities and how one may include them into daily life.
1. Echinacea (purpurea)

Overview: Considered the purple conefower, echinacea is among the most often used herb for immune support. Native Americans have long treated wounds and diseases using it.

advantages:

increases the activity of white blood cells—necessary for the fight against infections.

Lessens the severity and length of colds and other upper respiratory illnesses.

Comprising elements including polysaccharides, phenolic acids, and alkamides, which boost immune system,

One can take echinacea as a tablet, capsule, tincture, or tea. Starting echinacea at the first hint of illness and continuing for a few days after symptoms go away is advised most often.

Generally safe for temporary use. People allergic to the Asteraceae family—that is, ragweed, marigolds—should steer clear of echinacea.
2. Elderberry (Nigra sambucus)

Elderberry is a dark purple berries used historically to treat colds, flu, and other respiratory problems.

Drawbacks:

Packed in vitamins and antioxidants, including vitamin C, which boosts immune system.

Included are anthocyanins, anti-inflammatory and antiviral agents.

helps cut the length and intensity of flu and cold symptoms.

Elderberry is sold as a lozenge, gummy, syrup, and capsule. One can also make it into tea or infused with water.

Safety: Usually safe as advised. Raw elderberries, leaves, and stems have poisonous elements thus they should not be eaten.
3. Astragalus membranaceus, or stragalus

An ancient Chinese herb with immune-boosting and adaptogenic qualities is astragalus.

Advantages:

improves white blood cell production and activity, especially that of macrophages and natural killer cells.

Has immune function supporting polysaccharides, flavonoids, and saponins.

Helps guard against inflammation and oxidative stress.

One can have astragalus as a tea, tincture, capsule, or tablet. Traditionally Chinese medicine makes use of it in soups and broths.

Generally safe for long-term usage. Those with autoimmune illnesses should see a doctor before starting any treatment.
4. Garlic, or Allium sativum

Overview: Not only a common cooking tool but also a potent plant for immune support is garlic.

advantages:

includes allicin, a chemical having powerful immune-boosting and antibacterial action.

Indices the activity of immune cells including natural killer cells, lymphocytes, and macrophages.

Has antifungal, antibacterial, and antiviral properties.

Raw, cooked, or taken as a supplement— garlic can be eaten capsules or tablet form. Garlic's benefits are enhanced by crushing or chopping it then letting it sit for a few minutes before cooking.

Safety: Usually good for ingestion. Too much intake could upset the gut and interact with blood-thinning drugs.
5. Ginger, or Zingiber officinale.

Overview: Though it contains immune-boosting qualities, ginger is most well-known for its digestive aid.

Ad advantages:

Features gingerol, a bioactive chemical with anti-inflammatory and antioxidant properties.

aids to lower inflammation and improve immune system.

supports the respiratory system and eases flu and cold symptoms.

Ginger can be drank as a tea, fresh or dried, or as a supplement in capsules or pills. Cooking and baking also call for it somewhat frequently.

Safety: Generally speaking, for most people, rather safe. Overindulgence could lead to stomach trouble or heartburn.
6. Curcuma longa, or turmeric

Overview: Often found in Indian food and traditional medicine, turmeric is a vivid yellow spice.

Rewards:

Has curcumin, a chemical having strong anti-inflammatory and antioxidant action.

aids in immune system modulation and increases the body's capacity for infection fighting.

by lowering oxidative stress and inflammation supports general health.

Use: Turmeric can be used as a spice in cuisine, a drink, or as a supplement— capsules or tablets. Black pepper and turmeric together improve curcume absorption.

Safety: Generally speaking, for most people, rather safe. High doses could interfere with drugs meant to thin blood and create stomach problems.
7. holy basil (Ocimum sanctum)

Known by many as tulsi, holy basil is an adaptogenic herb prized in Ayurvedic medicine for its immune-supportive qualities.

Drawbacks:

increases the body's stress-resistance, therefore undermining the immune system.

Features eugenol, rosmarinic acid, and other substances bolstering immune system function.

has antioxidant, anti-inflammatory, and antibacterial qualities.

Holy basil may be taken as a supplement, tincture, or tea. Cooking and traditional medicine for some diseases also benefit from it.

Generally safe for most people. Those with specific medical issues should see a doctor prior to use.
8. Ginseng (Panax spp.).

For millennia, people have employed the adaptogenic plant ginseng to improve general energy and health.

Drawbacks:

aids in immune system modulation and enhancement of resistance against infections.

Contains ginsenosides, anti-inflammatory and immune-boosting agents.

Increases general energy levels and lessens tiredness.

Ginseng can be taken as a tincture, tea, capsule or tablet supplement. Traditional medicine frequently uses it to support general health.

Generally safe for most people. High doses might produce side effects including stomach discomfort, sleeplessness, and headache. Glycyrrhiza glabra, licorice root

Overview: Traditionally used as a plant with calming and immune-supportive qualities, licorice root is

Advantues:

Features glycyrrhizin, with antiviral and anti-inflammatory properties.

supports respiratory health and helps the immune system to be balanced.

eases coughing and other respiratory problems like sore throats.

Licorice root can be drank as a supplement, tincture, or tea. advised to avoid possible negative effects is deglycyrrhizinated licorice (DGL).

Generally safe for temporary use. High doses or continuous use can cause negative effects including potassium imbalances and high blood pressure.
10. Andrographis paniculata:

In traditional Asian medicine, andrographis is a herb frequently used to support immune system function.

Rewards:

Contains andrographolides, with anti-inflammatory, immune-boosting, antiviral action.

Lessens the severity and length of flu and colds.

Promotes respiratory health and general immune system.

Andrographis can be taken capsules or tablets or as a tincture or tea. It's frequently used to boost immune response at the first hint of disease.

Generally safe for temporary use. For some people, high doses could trigger allergic reactions and stomach trouble.

Remedies for Pain and Inflammation
Common diseases that could seriously affect quality of life are pain and

inflammation. Although traditional pharmaceuticals such as analgesics and nonsteroidal anti-inflammatory drugs (NSAIDs) are frequently used to treat these disorders, natural therapies can offer good and all-around substitutes. Key herbs and natural remedies with anti-inflammatory and pain-relieving qualities are included here.
1. Turmeric (longa Curcuma).

Overview: Often found in Indian food and traditional medicine, turmeric is a vivid yellow spice.

advantages:

Curcumin: Strong anti-inflammatory and antioxidant action characterizes the main component in turmeric. It lessens pain and blocks inflammatory processes.

Turmeric can help with muscle aches and injuries as well as joint pain and inflammation connected with arthritis.

Turmeric can be used as a spice in cuisine, a drink, or in supplement form—capsules or pills. Black pepper and turmeric together improve curcume absorption.

Safety: Generally speaking, for most people, rather safe. High doses could interfere with drugs meant to thin blood and create stomach problems.

2. Ginger (Zingiber officinale)

Overview: Though it has strong anti-inflammatory and pain-relieving qualities, ginger is most known for its digestive advantages.

Advantage:

The bioactive element in ginger, gingerol, has antioxidant and anti-inflammatory properties. It lowers pain and inflammation.

Ginger may aid with pain related to menstrual cramps, osteoarthritis, and muscular soreness.

Ginger can be drank as a tea, fresh or dried, or taken as a supplement in pills or capsules. Cooking and baking also call for it somewhat frequently.

Safety: Generally speaking, for most people, rather safe. Overindulgence could lead to stomach trouble or heartburn.

3. Boswellia serrata, or boswellia.

Extracted from the Boswellia tree, boswellia—also known as Indian frankincense—has been used for ages to relieve inflammation and discomfort.

Results:

By blocking inflammatory enzymes, boswellic acids—active substances—have great anti-inflammatory action.

Conditions such rheumatoid arthritis and osteoarthritis can cause pain and stiffness; boswellia can assist with both.

Boswellia is sold in pills, capsules, and topical lotions. Usually, a dosage ranges from 300 to 500 mg of standardized extract given two to three times daily.

Safety: Generally speaking, for most people, rather safe. There are those who might have stomach trouble.
4. Salix alba, white wither bark

Overview: Natural painkillers and anti-inflammatory agents have long come from white willow bark. It has a chemical akin to aspirin called salicin.

Ad advantages:

Salicin is turned in the body into salicylic acid, a substance with anti-inflammatory and analgesic effects.

White willow bark can assist with headaches, back discomfort, osteoarthritis, and menstrual cramps.

White willow bark can be taken as a tincture, pill, or tea depending on preferred form. Usually, a dosage ranges from 120 to 240 mg of salicin daily.

Safety: Generally speaking, for most people, rather safe. Those on blood-thinning drugs or those allergic to aspirin shouldn't use it.

5. Devil's Claw (Harpagophytum procumbens)

Native to southern Africa, devil's claw is a herb used historically to relieve inflammation and discomfort.

Ad advantages:

Harpagoside: Active in devil's claw, harpagoside possesses analgesic and anti-inflammatory properties.
Conditions include osteoarthritis, back discomfort, and tendonitis can all benefit from devil's claw's ability to help lower pain and inflammation.

Devil's claw comes in tinctues, capsules, and tablets. Usually, a dose ranges from 600 to 1,200 mg of extract given two to three times daily.

Safety: Generally speaking, for most people, rather safe. Those who have stomach ulcers or gallstones should avoid it since it could induce stomach pain.

6. Arnica (montana)

Overview: Topically utilized flowering plant arnis treats inflammation and pain.

Drawbacks:

Sesquiterpene lactones are analgesic and anti-inflammatory agents.

Arnica can help bruises, sprains, muscle pains, and arthritis-related pain and swelling go down.

Arnica finds frequent application in ointments, creams, and gel form. One shouldn't use it orally or on broken skin.

Safety: Usually rather safe for topical application. May irritate some people's skin.

7. Capsaicin (species of Capscium).

Overview: The active ingredient in chili peppers noted for their spiciness and pain-relieving qualities is capsaicin.

Ad advantages:

Capaicin acts by decreasing substance P,
a neuropeptide implicated in pain signal
transmission. It works well for lowering
pain from disorders like neuropathy,
arthritis, and muscular soreness.

Use: Capsaicin finds use in patches, gels,
and topical creams. It should be applied
as advised in the impacted region.

Usually safe for topical application.
Applied will give a burning sensation.
8. Ginger and Turmeric Mix

Combining turmeric and ginger might
improve their anti-inflammatory and
analgesic properties.

Rewards:

Curcumin and gingerol taken together
provide a strong anti-inflammatory and
analgesic action, which helps ailments
including arthritis and muscular
discomfort.

Use: The combo can be taken as a
supplement, in capsules, or as tea.
Taken twice daily, a normal dosage
consists in 500 milligrams of turmeric
and 500 mg of ginger extract.

Safety: Generally speaking, for most people, rather safe. Strong amounts could cause stomach problems.
9. Cloves (syzygium aromaticum)

Clove is a spice with known analgesic and anti-inflammatory qualities.

Benefits:

Strong anti-inflammatory and pain-relieving properties abound in the active element in clove, eugenol.

Clove oil can assist with toothache, sore gums, and muscle pain.

Use: Clove is a cooking, tea, and essential oil ingredient. A few drops of clove oil can be dabbed into a cotton ball and placed on the afflicted toothache site.

Generally safe for most people. Clove oil can irritate skin, hence one should use it carefully.
Ten: Rosemary, Rosmarinus officinalis

Rosemary is a plant often used in cooking but also possesses anti-inflammatory and pain-relieving qualities.

Advantues:

Rosmarinic Acid is a chemical having analgesic and anti-inflammatory properties.

Rosemary can assist with headaches, joint discomfort, and muscle pain.

Rosemary is a spice used in cooking, a tea, and an essential oil. Rosemary oil can be diluted with a carrier oil then applied to the afflicted area for topical treatment.

Safety: Generally speaking, for most people, rather safe. Overindulgence could lead to digestive problems.

Herbal Solutions for Skin Health
The biggest organ in the body, the skin protects it from outside factors. Not only for appearance but also for general health is maintaining good skin vital. Herbal treatments with their natural qualities and few side effects have been utilized for millennia to support skin condition. These are some important herbs well-known for improving skin condition, together with useful approaches to include them into your skincare regimen.
Aloe Vera (Aloe barbadensis miller)

Overview: Succulent and well-known for its healing and relaxing qualities is aloe vera.

Advantages:

Aloe vera gel helps to maintain skin hydration by being quite moistening.

Healing: It soothes burns, cuts, and abrasions, promotes healing of wounds.

Reducing inflammation and redness, anti-inflammatory agents help to treat sunburn and damaged skin.

Antimicrobial: Treats acne and helps ward against infections.

Aloe vera gel can be rubbed straight on skin. Many skincare products like lotions, creams, and masks also feature it. Most advantages come from fresh aloe gel straight from the plant.

Safety: Usually rather safe for topical application. A patch test is advised since some people could have allergic responses.
2. Calendula (officinalis calendula).

Traditionally, calendula—also called marigold—has been used to treat wounds and enhance skin condition.

Advantages:

Healing: Helps wounds to heal and lessens the scarring appearance.

Calms angry skin and lowers redness with anti-inflammatory action.

Antimicrobial: Treats mild illnesses and stops bacterial proliferation.

Moisturizing maintains silky, moisturized skin.

Calendula finds application in lotions, ointments, and infused oils. One can also use it as a skin's tea rinse.

Safety: Usually rather safe for topical application. People allergic to Asteraceae family plants should steer clear of calendula.
3. Lavender (Angustifolia angustifolia).

Lavender's soothing aroma and skin-healing qualities are well-known.

advantages:

Reducing inflammation and so calming inflamed skin helps.

By lowering bacterial count on the skin, antimicrobial helps treat and prevent acne.

Healing: Encouragement of cuts, burns, and other skin injuries' healing

Anti-aging: Features antioxidants meant to shield the skin from environmental harm and slow down aging's effects.

Use: Dilute lavender oil with a carrier oil then dab it over your skin. It also appears in facial sprays, creams, and lotions. One can use a toner from lavender-infused water.

Generally safe for topical application when diluted. May cause skin irritation in certain people; hence, a patch test is advised.

4. Alternifolia Tea Tree, Melaleuca

Overview: Renowned for its strong antibacterial and anti-inflammatory qualities, tea tree oil comes from the leaves of the tea tree.

Advantage:

Effective against viruses, bacteria, and fungi, antimicrobial agents help to treat skin infections including acne.

Reducing redness and inflammation linked with acne and other skin disorders, anti-inflammatory treatments

Healing: Encourages the tiny cuts, scratches, and bug bites to heal.

Before you apply tea tree oil to your skin, dilute it with a carrier oil. Additionally present in cleansers, toners, and acne spot treatments is it.

Usually safe for topical application when diluted. In some people, undiluted tea tree oil can irritate skin and set off allergic responses.

5. Chamomile (Matricaria chamomilla)

Chamomile is a common choice for sensitive skin since its anti-inflammatory and relaxing qualities are well-known.

Rewards:

Calms itchy and inflamed skin to suit disorders including eczema and dermatitis.

Antioxidant: guards against environmental harm to the skin.

Healing: Helps little cuts heal and lessens the look of scars.

Anti-inflammatory: lowers swelling and redness.

Uses include chamomile as an essential oil diluted with a carrier oil, in lotions, and as a tea rinse. One can use water enhanced with chamomiles as a toner.

Safety: Usually rather safe for topical application. Those allergic to Asteraceae family plants should steer clear of chamomile.

6. Witch Hazel (Hamamelis virginiana)

Long used in skincare for its astringent and anti-inflammatory qualities, witch hazel is a plant.

advantages:

For oily and acne-prone skin, astringent tones pores and lessens oiliness.

Anti-inflammatory: lowers redness and inflammation.

Treats mild skin irritations, bug bites, and sunburn.

Antioxidant: Shields the skin from environmental harm.

Use: Witch hazel can be used into lotions and creams or used as a toner. Over-the-counter astringents and cleansers frequently contain it.

Usually safe for topical application. Should be used sparingly since some people get dryness or discomfort from it. 7. Rosemary (Rosmarinus officinalis).

Overview: Although rosemary is a herb used often in cooking, it also has great effects on skin.

Advances:

Antioxidant: guards against environmental damage and aging's indicators on the skin.

Reduces redness and swelling: anti-inflammatory

Antimicrobial: Helps stop skin infections including acne.

Blood circulation is improved by which one promotes a good, radiant complexion.

Rosemary is included in skincare products including creams and serums or used as an essential oil diluted with a carrier oil. One uses a face rinse from rosemary-infused water.

Generally safe for topical application when diluted. May cause skin irritation in certain people; hence, a patch test is advised.

8. Neem (azadirachta indica)

Ayurvedic medicine makes great use of neem because of its broad spectrum of skin advantages.

Advantues:

Effective against viruses, bacteria, and fungi, antimicrobial agents help to treat skin infections including acne.

Reduces redness and inflammation: anti-inflammatory.

Healing: Helps little injuries heal and lessens scarring.

Moisturizing maintains the skin supple and hydrated.

Neem oil can be combined with a carrier oil or straight applied to the skin. Face masks and cleanses call for neem powder. Many skincaring products also contain neem.

Generally speaking, safety is high for topical application. May cause skin

irritation in certain people; hence, a patch test is advised.
9. Gotu Kola—Centella asiatica

Overview: Gotu kola's skin-healing qualities have long been sought for in traditional medicine.

Advantages:

Healing: Works to repair wounds and lessens the look of stretch marks and scars.

Reducing redness and inflammation, anti-inflammatory drugs help disorders including psoriasis and eczema.

Collagen synthesis is stimulated by this, therefore enhancing skin elasticity and firmness.

Antioxidant: guards against environmental harm to the skin.

Gotu kola can be extracted, used as a lotion or serum. Skincare products aimed at damaged and aging skin frequently feature it.

Usually safe for topical application. May cause skin irritation in certain people; hence, a patch test is advised.
10. Camellia sinensis, Green Tea

Overview: Green tea improves the skin extensively and is high in antioxidants.

Advantages:

Protects the skin from free radical damage and lessens aging symptoms by means of antioxidants.

Reduces redness and swelling, anti-inflammatory.

Antimicrobial: Helps stop skin infections including acne.

Offers some defense against UV damage.

Green tea is found in many skincare products, utilized in face masks, and a toner. Additionally found in serums and creams is green tea extract.

Safety: Usually rather safe for topical application. Most skin types accept green tea really nicely.

CHAPTER 5

Preparing and Using Herbal Remedies

For millennia, people from many civilizations have employed herbal treatments to treat different diseases and support general health. Knowing how to correctly make and use these treatments will help to guarantee safety and improve their potency. Together with excellent practices for including herbal treatments into your daily schedule, there is a thorough instruction on the several techniques of making and applying them.

1. Infusions and Herbal Teas

Herbal teas—also referred to as infusions—are among the easiest and most common uses for herbs. Infusions are hot water steeping of herbs' leaves, blossoms, or stems to release their medicinal ingredients.

How should one get ready?

Bring some fresh water to boil.

For every cup of water, use one to two teaspoon of dried herbs or two to three teaspoon of fresh herbs.

Steeping calls for filling a teapot or infuser with herbs, pouring boiling water over them, then covering. Depending on the herb and desired strength, let steep five to fifteen minutes.

Strain the herbs and drink your tea. If preferred, add honey or lemon for taste.

Herbs Perfect for Teas: echinacea, peppermint, ginger, lemon balm, chamomile.
Two: Decoctions

Overview: To extract their medicinal chemicals, decoctions boil harder plant elements including roots, bark, and seeds, much as infusions do.

How one should prepare?

To a pot, add one to two tablespoons of dried herbs per cup of water.

Bring to boil; then, lower the heat and simmer for 20 to 30 minutes.

Strain the liquid then savor your decoction. It can be drank cold or heated.

From ginger root to licorice root to dandelion root to cinnamon bark, best herbs for decoctions.
Three: Tinctures

Tinctues are concentrated herbal extracts created from soaking herbs in glycerin or alcohol. Comparatively to teas and decoctions, they are strong and have a longer shelf life.

How should one get ready?

Herbs and Alcohol: Halfway fill a glass jar with dry herbs (or three-quarters full with fresh herbs). Pour alcohol—such as brandy or vodka—over the herbs till well covered. glycerin for a non-alcoholic tincture.

Steeping: Seal the jar and keep it 4 to 6 weeks in a cold, dark environment. Daily shaking of the jar.

Strain the mixture through a fine-mesh strainer or cheese cloth following the steeping time. Bottle Stow the liquid in a dark glass bottle.

Usually taken in tiny amounts—one to two droppersful (20 to 40 drops) diluted in water or juice, two to three times a day.

Elderberries, ashwagandha, valerian root, echinacea—best herbs for tinctures.
4. Oils from Herbs

Herbal oils are created by herbs infusing carrier oils. Massage, skincare, and topical therapies all find use for them.

How would one prepare?

Herbs and Oil: Halfway fill a glass jar with dry herbs. Pour a carrier oil—such as olive oil, coconut oil, or jojoba oil—over the herbs until entirely covered.

Seal the jar and set it in a warm, sunny area for two to four weeks. Daily shaking of the jar.

Strain the oil through a fine-mesh strainer or cheese cloth following the infusion period. Bottle. For storage, move the oil to a fresh, dark glass bottle.

Herbal oils can be used in handcrafted salves and balms or straight on the skin.

Best Herbs for Oils: lavender, arnica, calendula, chamomile.
5. Uses & Balms Salves

Making salves and balms combines herbal oils with beeswalk or another thickening ingredient. Topically, they help to calm and repair the skin.

How best to get ready?

Melt one part beesw wax (or another thickening ingredient) with four parts herbal oil in a double boiler.

Once melted, toss the mixture into a clean container and allow it cool and set.

Essential oils are optional additions with extra therapeutic value.

Use salves and balms as advised for the afflicted skin area.

Comfrey, plantain, calendula, St. John's wort—best herbs for salves and balms.
6. Herbal powders and capsules.

Overview: For people who want not to drink teas or use tinctures, herbal capsules and powders are practical methods to take herbs.

How best to get ready?

Dust powdered herbs into empty capsules using a capsule machine. Use the machine's given directions.

Herbs can either bought pre-powdered or ground finely using a coffee grinder.

Use as directed by a healthcare professional or the advised dosage shown on the product label.

Among the best herbs for capsules and powders are turmeric, spirulina, moringa, and ashwagandha.

7. Herbal Comforts

Herbal compresses are soaking a cloth in a strong herbal infusion or decoction then rubbing it across the skin. They help healing, lower inflammation, and ease pain.

How would one prepare?

Prepare a strong infusion or decoction out of your selected plants.

Soak a fresh cloth or gauze in the herbal liquid, squeeze out the extra, and then apply it to the afflicted region. To hold heat, cover with a dry cloth.

Leave the compress on for fifteen to twenty minutes. As needed, repeat.

Among the best herbs for compresses are comfrey, chamomile, calendula, and witch hazel.

Eight: Herbal Steam Inhalation

Overview: Skin care and respiratory health benefit from steam inhalation including herbs. The steam helps the sinuses to be cleared and pores opened.

How should one get ready?

Boil water; then, pour it into a heat-safe bowl.

Add to the heated water a handful of fresh or dried herbs.

Lean over the bowl, cover your head with a towel to catch the steam, then inhale deeply five to ten minutes. Use great caution with the hot steam to prevent burns.

Eucalyptus, peppermint, rosemary, chamomile are best herbs for steam inhalation.

9. Herbal Baths

Herbal baths offer advantages for the psyche as well as the skin since they are soothing and healing.

How should I prepare?

Put one to two cups of dry herbs in a muslin bag or cheese cloth.

Fill the bathtub with hot water then submerge the bag of herbs such that it steeps for ten to fifteen minutes.

Take a 20 to 30 minute herbal bath. The heated water aids in the release of the herbs' helpful molecules.

Rose petals, lavender, chamomile, calendula are the best herbs for baths.

THE END

Made in the USA
Las Vegas, NV
23 December 2024

15246758R00037